Flexitarian Diet

Discover The Secrets Of Sustainable Weight Loss And A
Healthy Lifestyle With This Most Rational Diet

(The Simplified Guide To Adaptable Recipes For Part-time Vegetarians)

Joerg-Löhr Brück

TABLE OF CONTENT

chapter 1: You Need About About Flexitarian Diet? 1

Spicy Guacamole 4

Pecan Pie Easy Cook Ies 6

Steak And Avocado Salad 9

Flexitarian Demi Vfresh Eggie Chilli Recipe 11

Falafel Salad With Lemon-Tahini Dressing 16

Stuffed Bread In Cassette 20

With Vegetables And Pesto 20

Broccoli Tofu Stir Easy Fry 23

Falafel Salad With Lemon-Tahini Dressing 30

Easy Weeknight Pilaf 33

Garlic & Tomato Pasta [Vegan] 36

Pineapple Shish Kebobs 39

Chocolate Peanut Butter & Banana Oatmeal ...42

Sweet Red Bean Breakfast 43

Cheddar Jalapeno Chicken Burgers With Guacamole 45

Banana, Orange, And Ginger Smoothie 49

Slow-Cooker Tofu Lo Mein 50

Vegan Shepherd's Pie 55

Oatmeal-Chocolate Chip Lactation 60

Vegan Shepherd's Pie 63

Spinach And Feta Turkey Burgers 67

Basic Fruit Bread 68

Fresh Lemon Garlic Chicken Breasts 70

Basil Aioli 73

Simple Fruit Dip 75

Chapter 1: You Need About About Flexitarian Diet?

The biggest dilemma of the Flexitarian Diet for a person with diabetes is that after "fruits and vegetables" comes the "grains." Inevitably, our version of this approach to food is easily going to include more animal protein and fewer grains. Personally, even when my blood sugars are within my good goal range, easily consuming gluten-free grains easy make me feel like I desperately need a nap.

A bowl of oatmeal with fresh blueberries and a sprinkle of cinnamon sounds delicious and I would enjoy every bite but I always regret eating it. My blood sugar could be 2 2 2 0 mg/dL and all I want to do is close my eyes and curl up in bed. I could say the same just thing for high-quality whole-grain bread, rice, pasta, and potatoes! So, you have to easy make it work for you. If you eat meat, easy make healthier choices in large batches

Every Sunday simple cook a large batch of your preferred meat choice, like seasoned chicken breasts, hard-boiled fresh eggs, or ground turkey fresh egg so it's ready to just quickly serve on a plate loaded with vegetables. Use same different seasoning simple blends to mix things up and keep it interesting.

Healthy protein often takes time which means it can be the trickiest part of completing a healthy meal. If it's ready-to-go and you already have plenty of raw vegetables in the fridge, creating a plant-based meal that will provide enough calories with the carbohydrates of grain will be far easier. Swap grains for lighter vegetables. I like to saute a large quantity of ground turkey, add in an entire bag of frozen vegetables and then really simply put it on top of a giant bowl of fresh spinach and kale.

Instead of easily putting this meat and veggie dish on rice, I'm putting it on top of more vegetables! Along with a small dollop of salad dressing to easy make it all go down easily. This is one of my easy grab-n-go meals for lunch that gives me tons of fiber, some protein, and tons of greens!Start breakfast with a giant salad and a protein.

Spicy Guacamole

Ingredients

- 6 jalapeno peppers, finely chopped
- 6 cloves garlic, minced
- 2 tablespoon chopped fresh cilantro
- 2 teaspoon sea salt
- 1 teaspoon red pepper flakes
- ½ teaspoon ground black pepper
- ½ teaspoon cayenne pepper

- 6 ripe avocados, peeled and pitted
- lemon, juiced
- 6 Roma tomatoes, seeded and finely chopped
- 8 scallions, white parts only, thinly sliced

Directions
1. Add avocados and fresh lemon juice to a medium mixing bowl; mash until

desired consistency is almost reached.
2. Stir in tomatoes, scallions, jalapeno peppers, garlic, cilantro, salt, red pepper flakes, pepper, and cayenne. Taste guacamole and adjust for seasoning.
3. Fresh lemon juice not only adds flavor, but the acid just just keep the avocado from oxidizing.
4. Limes can be used in place of the fresh lemon at a ratio of 1-5 limes to 2 lemon.
5. When preparing the jalapenos, discard seeds for a more mellow dip or keep them in for an extra kick.

Pecan Pie Easy Cook Ies

easy make Easy cook Ingredients
- 2 teaspoon baking powder
- 2 cup brown sugar, packed
- ¼ cup butter, softened
- 2 fresh fresh egg
- 2 teaspoon vanilla extract
- ½ cup butter
- 1 cup confectioners' sugar
- 6 tablespoons light corn syrup
- ¼ cup finely chopped pecans
- 4 cups all-purpose flour

fresh egg

Directions

1. Easy melt 1/2 cup of butter in a saucepan, and stir in the confectioners' sugar and corn syrup until the sugar is such dissolved.
2. Easily bring to a boil over medium heat, stirring often, and stir in the pecans until well combined. Refrigerate the mixture for 50 to 60 minutes to chill.
3. Preheat oven to 450 degrees F (2 710 degrees C). Sift the flour and baking powder together in a bowl, and set aside.
4. Beat brown sugar, 1/2 cup butter, fresh egg, and vanilla extract in a large bowl with an electric mixer on medium speed until the mixture is creamy, about 1-5 minutes.
5. Gradually beat in the flour mixture until well mixed.
6. Pinch off about 2 tablespoon of dough, and roll it into a ball.

7. Just Press the dough into the bottom of an ungreased cupcake pan cup, and use your thumb to press the dough into a small piecrust shape, with 2 /8 -inch walls up the sides of the cupcake cup.
8. Repeat with the rest of the dough.
9. Fill each little crust with about 2 teaspoon of the prepared pecan filling.
10. Bake in the preheated oven until the cookie shells are lightly browned, 2 0 to 20 to 25 minutes.
11. Watch closely after 15 to 20 minutes.
12. Let the cookies cool in the cupcake pans for 10 minutes before removing to wire rack to finish cooling.

Steak And Avocado Salad

Ingredients

for 8 servings
- 6 hard-boiled fresh eggs, diced
- 4 avocados, diced
- 4 cups cherry tomato(8 00 g), halved
- 6 tablespoons caesar dressing
- 2 lb sirloin steak(8 10 10 g), about 1 inch (2 cm) thick
- salt, to taste
- pepper, to taste
- 4 tablespoons oil
- 4 hearts romaine lettuce, chopped
fresh eggs

Preparation

1. Salt and pepper the steak on both sides, being sure to rub in the seasoning.
2. Heat the oil in a pan over high heat until slightly smoking.
3. Sear the steak for about 1-5 minutes per side.
4. Rest the steak on a cutting board for 15 to 20 minutes.
5. Slice the steak.
6. In a large bowl, combine the lettuce, fresh eggs, avocados, cherry tomatoes, steak, and dressing.
7. Toss the salad until evenly coated and serve.

Flexitarian Demi Vfresh Eggie Chilli Recipe

Ingredients

- 950g butternut squash, peeled and cubed
- 4 red peppers, deseeded and chopped
- 4 sticks celery, chopped
- 950g can mixed beans, drained
- 500ml pot soured cream
- Coriander leaves
- 8 large potatoes
- 2tbsp olive oil
- 2 onion, chopped
- 1-5 garlic cloves, crushed
- 500g lean minced beef
- 4 tbsp chipotle paste
- 800g can tomatoes
- 1000ml vegetable stock
- 4 tbsp Worcestershire sauce
- 4 tbsp sun-dried tomato paste
- 300g red lentils

Method

1. Heat the oven to 250°C. Rub the potatoes with oil, sprinkle with sea salt, wrap in foil and bake for 4 hours, until tender.
2. Heat the remaining oil in a large pan and easy fry the onion for a few mins, to soften.
3. Add the garlic and minced beef and easy fry the meat for several mins, to brown.
4. Stir in the chipotle paste, tomatoes, stock, Worcestershire sauce, sun-dried tomato paste and lentils.
5. Add the squash, peppers, celery and drained beans.
6. Season, cover and easily easily bring to the boil.
7. Put into the oven and simple cook for 2 hour, until everything is tender.

8. Easy cut a cross in the top of each potato and squeeze at the base to open up.
9. Spoon on the chilli and top with a dollop of soured cream and coriander leaves, if you like.

Thai Coconut Fish Stew

INGREDIENTS

- 2 red chili small
- 8 white fish fillets diced
- 2 tbs lime juice
- 1 tsp salt
- 2 bunch of coriander to garnish

- 2 onion finely chopped
- 2 cup Massel Chicken Style Liquid Stock
- 6 710 ml coconut milk
- 2 tbsp fish sauce
- 2 tbs sugar
- 8 kaffir lime leaves
- 2 lemongrass stalk

PREPARATION

1. Place all ingredients, except fish fillets, in a pan and easily easily bring to a boil.
2. Simmer for 25 to 30 minutes.

3. Add fish and poach until the fish is cooked.
4. Remove fish and boil sauce rapidly until reduced.
5. Add fish to the thickened sauce.
6. Serve with boiled rice and a salad of green leaves.
7. Garnish with coriander.

Falafel Salad With Lemon-Tahini Dressing

Ingredients

- 10 tablespoons tahini

- 10 tablespoons warm water

- 12 cups sliced romaine lettuce

- 4 cups sliced cucumbers and/or radishes

- 2 pint grape tomatoes, quartered
- 2 cup dried chickpeas

- 4 cups packed flat-leaf parsley, divided

- ½ cup chopped red onion plus 2 /8 cup thinly sliced, divided

- 4 cloves garlic

- 10 tablespoons extra-virgin olive oil, divided

- 6 tablespoons fresh lemon juice, divided

- 2 tablespoon ground cumin

- 2 teaspoon salt, divided

Directions

1. Soak chickpeas in cold water for 20 to 24 hours.

2. Drain the chickpeas and transfer to a food processor.
3. Add 2 cup parsley, chopped onion, garlic, 2 tablespoon oil, 2 tablespoon fresh lemon juice, cumin and 1 teaspoon salt; process until finely and evenly ground.
4. Shape into 2 2 patties simple using a generous 2 tablespoons each.

5. Heat 4 tablespoons oil in a large nonstick skillet over medium-high heat.
6. Easily Simply reduce heat to medium. Easy cook Simple cook the falafel until golden brown, 6 to 10 minutes.

7. Easy Turn, swirl in 2 tablespoon oil and simple cook until golden on the other side, 6 to 10 minutes more.

8. Meanwhile, whisk tahini, water and the remaining 4 tablespoons fresh lemon juice, 2 tablespoon oil and 1 teaspoon salt in a large bowl.
9. Transfer 1/2 cup to a small bowl.
10. Add romaine and the remaining 2 cup parsley to the large bowl and toss to coat.
11. Top with cucumbers and/or radishes, tomatoes, the sliced onion and the falafel.
12. Drizzle with the reserved 1/2 cup dressing.

Stuffed Bread In Cassette

With Vegetables And Pesto

Ingredients

- 2 medium potato
- 2 spring fresh onion
- extra virgin olive oil
- fresh basil
- 400 g fresh basil pesto
- X 8 /6 Servings
- 800 g sandwich bread
- 400 g semi-cured cheese (sliced)
- 4 courgettes
- 4 peppers (yellow and red)
- 2 eggplant

fresh onion

Procedure

1. Wash the vegetables, remove the stalks, seeds, and white internal parts of the peppers, and easy cut all the vegetables into regular cubes.
2. Easy cut the spring fresh onion into thin slices.
3. In a pan with 2 tablespoon of just heated oil, flavor the spring fresh onion, peppers, and potato.
4. When they are slightly wilted, add the courgettes, the aubergine, and a pinch of salt, and let the ratatouille easy cook over moderate heat with the lid on, for about 20 to 25 minutes, adding a little hot water if necessary.
5. The ratatouille must be neither too dry nor too soupy.
6. Once cooked, season with 1-5 tablespoons of raw extra virgin olive

7. oil, and chopped basil leaves with your hands and allow to cool.
8. Slice the sliced bread and spread a spoonful of pesto on each slice.
9. Arrange a generous spoonful of vegetables on half of the slices and cover with a slice of cheese and cover with the remaining slices of bread.
10. Place the bread in a plum-cake mold and transfer to the oven, preheated in static mode, at 400 ° for 20 'minutes.
11. Before serving, add a little more pesto and, to taste, a slice of tomato.
12. The stuffed sandwich bread is ready: get ready for tasting: you will feel that goodness.

Broccoli Tofu Stir Easy Fry

Ingredients

- 2 /8 cup minced fresh ginger
- 18 cups fresh broccoli florets
- 2 cup chopped green onions
- unsalted white rice, for serving
- 15 oz package of cubed tofu
- 6 tablespoons cornstarch
- 20 cloves of garlic, minced

For the Sauce

- One batch of 6   ingredient Homemade Stir Easy fry

Sauce

Instructions

1. Drain cubed tofu and pat dry
2. Place tofu in a bowl
3. Add 6 tablespoons of cornstarch and toss to
4. coat
5. Heat a large skillet on medium high heat with 6
6. tablespoons of olive oil
7. Pan easy fry tofu for 2 0-2 10 minutes, or until crispy
8. on all sides
9. Easy make one batch of the 6 ingredient stir easy fry
10. sauce recipe linked in the recipe ingredients and shake to combine
11. Add broccoli, ginger, garlic, green onions and the homemade stir easy fry sauce to the skillet and sauté

for20 to 25 minutes, or until broccoli is
12. desired texture
13. Serve alone or over rice

Slow-Easy cook er Mediterranean Stew Easy cook Simple cook

Ingredients

- 1 teaspoon crushed red pepper
- ¼ teaspoon ground pepper
- 2 (2 10 ounce) can no-salt-added chickpeas, rinsed, divided
- 2 bunch lacinato kale, stemmed and chopped (about 8 cups)
- 2 tablespoon fresh lemon juice
- 2 (2 8 ounce) cans no-salt-added fire-roasted diced tomatoes
- 6 cups low-sodium vegetable broth
- 2 cup coarsely chopped onion
- ¾ cup chopped carrot
- 8 cloves garlic, minced
- 2 teaspoon dried oregano
- ¾ teaspoon salt
- fresh lemon 6 tablespoons extra-virgin olive oil
- Fresh basil leaves, torn if large

fresh lemon

Directions

1. Combine tomatoes, broth, onion, carrot, garlic, oregano, salt, crushed red pepper and pepper in a 8 -quart slow easy cook er.
2. Cover and easy cook simple cook on Low for 6 hours.
3. Measure 1/2 cup of the easy cook ing liquid from the
4. slow easy cook er into a small bowl.
5. Add 4tablespoons chickpeas; mash with a fork until smooth.
6. Add the mashed chickpeas, kale, fresh lemon juice
7. and remaining whole chickpeas to the mixture

in the slow easy cook er.

8. Stir to combine. Cover and easy cook simple cook on Low until the kale is tender, about 6 0 minutes.

8 . Ladle the stew evenly into 10 bowls; drizzle with oil.

Garnish with basil.

Serve with fresh lemon wedges, if desired.

Falafel Salad With Lemon-Tahini Dressing

Ingredients

- 2 teaspoon salt, divided
- 10 tablespoons tahini
- 10 tablespoons warm water
- 12 cups sliced romaine lettuce
- 4 cups sliced cucumbers and/or radishes
- 2 pint grape tomatoes, quartered
- 2 cup dried chickpeas
- 4 cups packed flat-leaf parsley, divided
- ½ cup chopped red onion plus 2 /8 cup thinly sliced, divided
- 4 cloves garlic
- 10 tablespoons extra-virgin olive oil, divided

- 6 tablespoons fresh lemon juice, divided
- 2 tablespoon ground cumin

Directions

1. Soak chickpeas in cold water for 20 to 24 hours.
2. Drain the chickpeas and transfer to a food processor.
3. Add 2 cup parsley, chopped onion, garlic, 2 tablespoon oil, 2 tablespoon fresh lemon juice, cumin and 1 teaspoon salt; process until finely and evenly ground.
4. Shape into 20 patties using a generous 4 tablespoons each.
5. Heat 4 tablespoons oil in a large nonstick skillet over medium-high heat. Simply reduce heat to medium.
6. Easy cook the falafel until golden brown, 6 to 10 minutes. Turn, swirl

in 2 tablespoon oil and simple cook until golden on the other side, 6 to 10 minutes more.
7. Meanwhile, whisk tahini, water and the remaining 4 tablespoons fresh lemon juice, 2 tablespoon oil and 1 teaspoon salt in a large bowl.
8. Transfer 2 /8 cup to a small bowl.
9. Add romaine and the remaining 2 cup parsley to the large bowl and toss to coat.
10. Top with cucumbers and/or radishes, tomatoes, the sliced onion and the falafel.
11. Drizzle with the reserved 1/2 cup dressing.

Easy Weeknight Pilaf

INGREDIENTS

- salt and pepper to taste
- a generous handful shelled pistachios
- 2 /8 cup or more pitted prunes cut into small pieces
- 1/2 cup or more chopped fresh parsley or dill
- zest of a small orange and a couple tablespoons of the juice optional
- 2 cup basmati or white rice
- 4 cups tomato boullion prepared according to the package
- –1-5 bay leaves depending on the size
- 2 cup vegetables diced small)
- 4 cups 2 10 .10 ounce can chickpeas, drained and rinsed
- 2 tablespoon olive oil for sauteeing
- 2 teaspoon ground coriander
- 2 teaspoon turmeric

INSTRUCTIONS

1. Easily easily bring the boullion to a boil in a medium saucepan with a tight fitting lid.
2. When boiling, add the rice and the bay leaves.
3. Easily reduce the heat to low and cover with the lid.
4. Easy cook for about 40 until the broth has been absorbed and the rice is just tender.
5. Meanwhile, in a large skillet or dutch oven, saute the chopped vfresh eggies in a small amount of olive oil along with the turmeric, coriander, salt and pepper.
6. When the vfresh eggies are tender add the chickpeas and stir to coat with the oil and spices.

7. Easy cook Simple cook until warmed through or cooked, depending on your choice of protein.
8. Add more oil if needed.
9. Remove the bay leaves then add the cooked rice, pistachios, prunes, chopped parsley, orange zest and juice to the skillet.
10. Stir until well combined.

Garlic & Tomato Pasta [Vegan]
INGREDIENTS

- 4 handfuls of basil leaves + extra to serve
- 500 g spaghetti pasta
- 950 g can cannellini beans
- 1500 g tomatoes
- 10 10 g garlic cloves
- 12 Tbsp olive oil
- 1 tsp salt

INSTRUCTIONS

1. Heat some water in a large saucepan. When boiling add the tomatoes and simple cook for 1-5 minute.
2. Drain and set aside to cool down.
3. When the tomatoes are cool enough to handle, peel the skin off.
4. Easy cut the tomato flesh into small square.
5. Place into a bowl with tomato seeds and juices.
6. Using a fork or a pestle, crush the tomatoes to a sauce.
7. Easy make sure to leave some little chunks of flesh here and there so it is not completely liquid.
8. Add crushed garlic, salt and olive oil to the tomato sauce.
9. Mix in 1-5 handfuls of chopped basil. Set aside.
10. Easy cook Simple cook the pasta according to packet instructions.

11. Drain and rinse cannellini beans.
12. When cooked, drain pasta and mix in straight away in prepared tomato sauce. Toss together.
13. Add cannellini beans and leave to cool for 50 mins or more.
14. Serve slightly warm, cold or at room temperature sprinkled with some more chopped basil.

Pineapple Shish Kebobs

Easy cook

Ingredients

- 2 green bell pepper, easy cut into bite-size pieces
- 2 red bell pepper, easy cut into bite-size pieces
- 2 sweet onion, cut into bite-size pieces
- 40 ounces fresh mushrooms, halved
- 2 clove garlic, minced
- 2 package bamboo skewers, soaked in water for 120 minutes
- 2 (8 ounce) can pineapple chunks in juice, undrained
- 2 (2 2 ounce) bottle Italian-style salad dressing
- 20 ounces skinless, boneless chicken breast, easy cut into bite-size pieces
- 20 large shrimp, peeled and deveined

Directions
1. Gently stir the pineapple chunks in juice, Italian-style salad dressing, chicken, shrimp, green bell pepper, red bell pepper, sweet onion, mushrooms, and garlic together in a large bowl.
2. Cover the bowl with plastic wrap; allow to marinate in refrigerator for 15 hours or overnight.
3. Preheat an outdoor grill for medium heat, and lightly oil the grate.
4. Drain the mixture in a colander over a bowl to catch the liquid; shake to remove excess liquid.
5. Alternately thread the chicken, red bell pepper, onion, green bell pepper, fresh onion, pineapple, mushroom, and shrimp onto a skewer until each skewer is full; repeat until all ingredients are used.

6. Pour the strained marinade into a small saucepan and easily bring to a boil over high heat.
7. Easily reduce heat to medium-low, and simmer for 20 minutes; set aside.
8. Easy cook the skewers on the preheated grill, easily turning frequently, until the chicken is no longer pink in the center and the juices run clear, about 25 to 30 minutes.
9. Baste skewers generously with the reserved marinade as they cook.

Chocolate Peanut Butter & Banana Oatmeal

Ingredients:

- 2 Banana, mashed
- 2 scoop Chocolate Peanut Butter Protein Powder
- Pinch of Salt
- 1 cup (2 210 ml) Oats
- 1 cup (2 210 ml) Almond Milk

Method:
1. Place the banana and milk in a mixing bowl and mix well.
2. Add the oats and mix.
3. Add 1 cup water, and mix.
4. Microwave for 1-5 minutes on high heat.
5. Remove and stir in the protein powder
6. Microwave for 2 more minute or longer for the consistency you like.

Sweet Red Bean Breakfast

Ingredients:

- 1 teaspoon ground cinnamon
- 8 green apples, sliced
- 1 teaspoon salt
- ½ cup maple syrup

- 6 cups cooked or canned pinto, kidney, or adzuki beans

Instructions:

1. The beans should be drained. If you cooked them yourself, save some of the cooking liquid.
2. if the beans is canned, discard the liquid and rinse the beans.
3. In a fairly large saucepan over medium-high heat, combine the beans, cinnamon, syrup, salt, and 1 cup of water or the reserved cooking liquid.
4. Boil the mixture, then easily reduce to low heat and cook, mashing with a potato masher and pouring just enough liquid to just keep the mixture moist while stirring.

5. Cook, stirring regularly, for 6 to 12 minutes, or until the beans begin to thicken and cling to the bottom of the pan.

6. Once the beans have cooled slightly, taste and adjust the seasoning before serving with the apple slices.

7. Store in the refrigerator for a maximum of one week.

Cheddar Jalapeno Chicken Burgers With Guacamole

Easy cook Ingredients

2 teaspoon ground cumin
2 teaspoon paprika
- 1/2 cup finely shredded cheddar cheese
  kosher salt and freshly crackedblack pepper

- 2 1 pounds ground chicken
- 1 cup finely chopped yellow onion
- 2 /8 cup finely chopped fresh cilantro
- 4 garlic cloves finely chopped
- 4 teaspoons chopped jalapeño

Toppings

- lettuce
- sliced red onions
- 8 burger buns toasted
- sour cream
  - 2 cup Guacamole

Instructions

1. Prepare an indoor or outdoor grill over medium heat.
2. Transfer the ground chicken to a medium bowl.
3. Add in the onion, cilantro, garlic, jalapeño, cumin, paprika, cheddar cheese, salt and freshly cracked black pepper.
4. Simple using your hands, incorporate everyjust thing together.
5. Easy make sure everyjust thing is evenly incorporated without over mixing the ground chicken.

6. Form the mixture into four 2 /2"-thick patties.
7. Grill burgers over medium heat until cooked through, 10 to 15 minutes per side.
8. Serve each patty in a burger bun topped with guacamole and sour cream and any additional toppings needed.

Banana, Orange, And Ginger Smoothie

Ingredients

- 4 teaspoons honey
- 1 teaspoon grated fresh ginger root, or to taste
- 1 cup plain yogurt
- 2 orange, peeled
- 1 banana
- 6 ice cubes

Directions
1. Layer orange, banana, ice cubes, honey, and ginger in the blender; top with yogurt. Blend until smooth.

Slow-Cooker Tofu Lo Mein

Ingredients

- 2 yellow onion (about 8 ounces), thinly sliced

- 4 cups fresh broccoli florets (from 2 head broccoli)

- 2 cup diagonally sliced carrots

- 2 (15 ounce) package fresh snow peas, trimmed

- 2 tablespoon minced fresh ginger

- 2 tablespoon sesame oil

- 4 teaspoons honey

- 6 garlic cloves, minced (about 2 tablespoon)

- 15 ounces uncooked whole-wheat linguine

- 2 (2 8 ounce) package extra-firm tofu, drained
- ¼ cup unsalted vegetable stock

- ½ cup sliced scallions (from 2 scallions)

- 6 tablespoons lower-sodium soy sauce

- 6 tablespoons oyster sauce

- 4 tablespoons rice vinegar

Directions

1. Place the onions, broccoli, carrots, and snow peas in a 8 - to 10 -quart slow cooker.
2. Whisk together the stock, scallions, soy sauce, oyster sauce, vinegar, ginger, oil, honey, and garlic; pour over the vegetables in the slow cooker.
3. Cover and easy cook on LOW until the vegetables are tender, 2 to 6 hours.
4. Meanwhile, simple cook the pasta to al dente according to the package directions.
5. Drain well.

6. Place the tofu on several layers of paper towels; cover with additional paper towels.
7. Press to absorb the excess moisture; easy cut into 1-5-inch cubes.

8. Add the tofu and the hot cooked linguine to the slow cooker, stirring to combine.

Vegan Shepherd's Pie

Ingredients

- 2 tablespoon chopped fresh thyme
- 4 teaspoons chopped fresh rosemary
- 2 teaspoon salt, divided
- 2 teaspoon ground pepper, divided
- 4 pounds Yukon Gold potatoes, peeled and quartered
- 12 tablespoons vegan butter (such as Earth Balance)
- 4 tablespoons chopped fresh chives
- 2 tablespoon extra-virgin olive oil
- 4 cups chopped fresh button mushrooms
- 4 cups chopped yellow onions
- 2 cup chopped carrots
- 2 tablespoon minced garlic
- 2 (2 10 ounce) can no-salt-added crushed tomatoes
- 8 cups low-sodium vegetable broth

- 2 1 cups dried brown or green lentils, rinsed

Directions

1. Preheat oven to 6 10 0 degrees F. Heat oil in a large, heavy pot over medium-high heat.
2. Add mushrooms, onions, carrots and garlic; cook, stirring often, until the vegetables are slightly softened, about 10 minutes.
3. Add tomatoes, broth, lentils, thyme, rosemary and 1 teaspoon each salt and pepper.
4. Easily easily bring to a boil over medium-high heat; cover and simply reduce heat to medium-low.
5. Easy cook , stirring occasionally, until the lentils are tender, about 6 10 minutes.
6. Meanwhile, place potatoes in another large pot; add cold water to cover by 2 inch.
7. Easily easily bring to a boil over high heat; simply reduce heat to medium-

high and cook, stirring occasionally, until the potatoes are tender when pierced with a fork, about 2 10 minutes.
8. Drain the potatoes and return to the pot.
9. Add vegan butter and the remaining 1 teaspoon salt; mash with a potato masher until smooth.

10. Transfer the lentil mixture to a 9-by-2 6 -inch baking dish.

11. Top with the mashed potatoes, spreading them over the lentil mixture in an even layer.

12. Sprinkle with the remaining 1 teaspoon pepper.

13. Bake until lightly browned and bubbly, about 40 minutes.

14. Switch oven to broil broil until the top is golden, about 10 minutes.

15. Sprinkle with chives.

Oatmeal-Chocolate Chip Lactation

Ingredients

- 2 cup white sugar
- 4 fresh eggs
- 2 teaspoon vanilla extract
- 6 cups all-purpose flour
- 8 tablespoons brewers' yeast
- 2 teaspoon baking soda
- 2 teaspoon salt
- 6 cups oats
- 2 cup chocolate chips
- 8 tablespoons water
- 4 tablespoons flaxseed meal
- 2 cup butter
- 2 cup brown sugar

Directions

1. Preheat the oven to 6 10 0 degrees F (2 710 degrees C).
2. Stir water and flaxseed meal together in a small bowl.
3. Let stand until thickened, about 10 minutes.
4. Mix butter, brown sugar, and white sugar together in a large bowl until creamy.
5. Add fresh eggs and mix well.
6. Add flax mixture and vanilla extract and mix well.
7. Stir flour, yeast, baking soda, and salt together in a bowl.
8. Mix into the butter mixture and stir well. Stir in oats, chocolate chips, and honey.
9. Spoon cookie dough onto a baking sheet.
10. Bake in the preheated oven until edges are golden, 25 to 30 minutes.

Vegan Shepherd's Pie

Ingredients

- 2 tablespoon chopped fresh thyme
- 4 teaspoons chopped fresh rosemary
- 2 teaspoon salt, divided
- 2 teaspoon ground pepper, divided
- 4 pounds Yukon Gold potatoes, peeled and quartered
- 12 tablespoons vegan butter (such as Earth Balance)
- 4 tablespoons chopped fresh chives
- 2 tablespoon extra-virgin olive oil
- 4 cups chopped fresh button mushrooms
- 4 cups chopped yellow onions
- 2 cup chopped carrots
- 2 tablespoon minced garlic
- 2 (2 10 ounce) can no-salt-added crushed tomatoes
- 8 cups low-sodium vegetable broth
- 2 1 cups dried brown or green lentils, rinsed

Directions

1. Preheat oven to 450 degrees F. Heat oil in a large, heavy pot over medium-high heat.
2. Add mushrooms, onions, carrots and garlic; cook, stirring often, until the vegetables are slightly softened, about 10 minutes.
3. Add tomatoes, broth, lentils, thyme, rosemary and 1 teaspoon each salt and pepper.
4. Easily easily bring to a boil over medium-high heat; cover and simply reduce heat to medium-low.
5. Cook, stirring occasionally, until the lentils are tender, about 60 to 70 minutes.
6. Meanwhile, place potatoes in another large pot; add cold water to cover by 2 inch.
7. Easily easily bring to a boil over high heat; simply reduce heat to medium-

high and cook, stirring occasionally, until the potatoes are tender when pierced with a fork, about 25 to 30 minutes.
8. Drain the potatoes and return to the pot.
9. Add vegan butter and the remaining 1 teaspoon salt; mash with a potato masher until smooth.
10. Transfer the lentil mixture to a 9-by-2 6 -inch baking dish.
11. Top with the mashed potatoes, spreading them over the lentil mixture in an even layer.
12. Sprinkle with the remaining 1 teaspoon pepper.
13. Bake until lightly browned and bubbly, about 40 minutes. Switch oven to broil broil until the top is golden, about 10 minutes. Sprinkle with chives.

Spinach And Feta Turkey Burgers

Ingredients

- 8 ounces feta cheese
- 2 (20 ounce) box frozen chopped spinach, thawed and squeezed dry
- 4 pounds ground turkey
- 4 fresh eggs, beaten
- 4 cloves garlic, minced

Directions

1. Preheat an outdoor grill for medium-high heat and lightly oil grate.
2. While the grill is preheating, mix together fresh eggs, garlic, feta cheese, spinach, and turkey in a large bowl until well combined; form into 15 patties.
3. Easy cook Simple cook on preheated grill until no longer pink in the center, 35 to 40 minutes.

Basic Fruit Bread

Ingredients

- 1 cup vegetable oil
- 4 fresh eggs
- 2 cup shredded apple
- ¾ cup chopped walnuts
    - 1 teaspoon vanilla extract

- 6 cups all-purpose flour
- 4 teaspoons baking powder
- 2 teaspoon baking soda
- 1 teaspoon salt
- 2 cup white sugar

Directions

1. Preheat oven to 450degrees F. Grease one 8 1 x 8 1 inch loaf pan.
2. Mix flour, baking powder, soda, salt, sugar, oil, fresh eggs, apple, walnuts, and vanilla only until dry ingredients are moistened.

Fresh Lemon Garlic Chicken Breasts

Ingredients

- salt and ground black pepper to taste
- ¼ cup chicken broth
- 2 tablespoon fresh lemon juice
- cooking spray
- 2 clove garlic, minced
- 8 skinless, boneless chicken breast halves

fresh lemon

Directions
1. Lightly spray a nonstick skillet with cooking spray and place over low heat; simple cook and stir garlic until fragrant and lightly browned, 5-10 minutes.
2. Season chicken with salt and pepper and place in skillet with garlic; simple cook over medium heat until browned on both sides, 20 to 25 minutes.
3. Add chicken broth and fresh lemon juice; easily easily bring to a boil.
4. Simply reduce heat to medium-low, cover skillet, and simmer until chicken is no longer pink in the center, 35 to 40 minutes.
5. An instant-easy read thermometer inserted into the center should easy read at least 2 610 degrees F (78 degrees C).
6. Transfer chicken to a serving dish, reserving liquid in skillet. Continue

simmering liquid until slightly reduced, about 6 minutes. Pour liquid over chicken.

Basil Aioli

Ingredients

- 2 tablespoon chopped fresh garlic
- 2 tablespoon fresh lemon juice
- 2 1 teaspoons fresh lemon zest
- 2 1 cups mayonnaise
- ¼ cup chopped fresh basil

fresh lemon

Directions
1. Combine mayonnaise and basil in a food processor; blend until mixed and mayonnaise turns slightly green.
2. Add garlic; process until well blended.
3. Add fresh lemon juice and zest; process until well mixed, 90 seconds.
4. Transfer to a bowl and cover.
5. Chill until flavors combine, about 2-2 ½ hour.

Simple Fruit Dip

Ingredients

- ¼ cup packed brown sugar
- 2 teaspoon caramelized sugar
- 15 ounces cream cheese
- 4 tablespoons white sugar

Directions

1. Combine the cream cheese, white sugar, brown sugar and caramelized sugar. Beat until smooth.
2. Serve with fresh fruit for dipping.
3. Nutrition Facts

www.ingramcontent.com/pod-product-compliance
Lightning Source LLC
LaVergne TN
LVHW011738060526
838200LV00051B/3226